PLANT-BASED COOKBOOK
FOR EVERYDAY COOKING

*50 Healthy and Delicious Plant-Based
Recipes Step to Step You'll Make Again
and Again*

Botanika Green Way

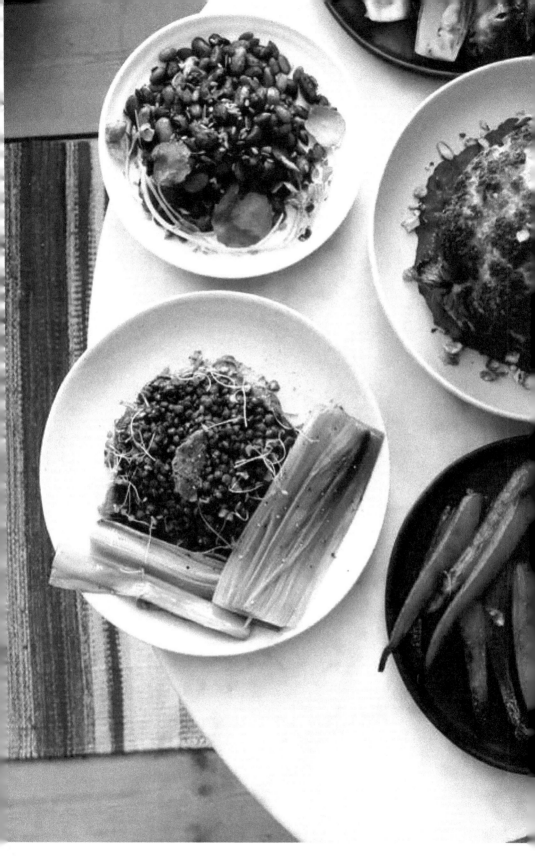

Table of Contents

INTRODUCTION

A plant-based diet is a diet based primarily on whole plant foods. Hence, it excludes animal-sourced foods, hydrogenated oils, refined sugars, and processed foods. A whole food plant-based diet does not consist solely of fruits and vegetables. It includes unprocessed or barely processed oils with healthy fats like extra-virgin olive oil, whole grains, legumes, seeds, and nuts, as well as herbs and spices.

What is the Plant-Based Diet?

The plant-based diet may seem similar to a vegetarian or vegan diet, but it is neither. It's not a diet but a healthy lifestyle. It uses food from plants, and it excludes processed foods like white rice and added sugars, which are allowed in vegan and vegetarian diets.

A plant-based diet is not a diet; it's a healthy way of life

The secret to a healthy diet is simpler than you ever thought! When following a plant-based dietary regimen, you should focus on plant-based foods and avoid animal-sourced food. Whether you are already following a vegan diet or are considering trying this lifestyle, this plant-based, budget-friendly food list makes your grocery shopping easy to manage.

- **VEGETABLES**

Try to include different types of vegetables in your diet from above-ground vegetables to root vegetables, which grow underground.

- **FRUITS**

Choose affordable fruits that are in season. Add frozen fruit to your grocery list since they are just as nutritious as fresh produce. They can be used in smoothies, toppings, compotes, or preserves. On the other hand, dried fruit generally contains a lot of antioxidants, especially polyphenols. It has been proven that eating dried fruits can prevent heart disease and some types of cancer.

- **NUTS & SEEDS**

Nuts and seeds offer different dietary benefits. They do not only ensure essential nutrients but are also offer a variety of flavors. This "ready to eat" food is a perfect snack with dried fruits and trail mix, essential vegan foods to stockpile for an emergency.

- **RICE & GRAINS**

Rice and grains are versatile and easy to incorporate into your diet. Leftovers reheat wonderfully and can be served at any time of the day, turning simple and inexpensive ingredients into a full-fledged meal. You can also make healthy nut butters such as tahini or peanut butter.

- **BEANS & LEGUMES**

Legumes and beans are highly affordable, and there's no end to the variety of tasty dishes you can cook with them. These humble but powerful foods are packed with vitamins, minerals, protein, and dietary fiber. In addition to being super-healthy and versatile, legumes pair very well with other proteins, vegetables, and grains.

- **HEALTHY FATS**

Don't underestimate the importance of quality fats in cooking. Coconut oil, olive oil, and avocado are always good to have on hand.

- **NON-DAIRY PRODUCTS**

Using a plant-based cheese or milk lends flavor, texture, and nutrition to your meals. You can find fantastic products on the market, and this book has many wonderful recipes for feta, vegan ricotta, and plant-based milk.

- **HERBS, SPICES & CONDIMENTS**

A handful of fresh herbs will add that little something extra to your soups, stews, dips, or casseroles. Condiments such as mustard, ketchup, vegan mayonnaise, and plant-based sauces can be used in salads, casseroles, and spreads. Choosing their distinctive flavors to complement vegetables, grains and legumes will help you to make the most of your vegan dishes. Herbs and spices are naturally plant-based, but play it safe and look for a label that says *Vegan-friendly*.

- **BAKING GOODS & CANNED GOODS**

These vegan essentials include all types of flour, baking powder, baking soda, and yeast. Further, cocoa powder, vegan chocolate, and sweeteners are good to have on hand. As for the healthy vegan sweeteners, opt for fresh or dried fruits, agave syrup, maple syrup, and stevia. When it comes to canned goods, stock your pantry with cooking essentials such as tomato, sauerkraut, pickles, low sodium chickpeas and beans, coconut milk, green chilies, pumpkin puree, tomato sauce, low sodium corn, and artichoke hearts. Thus, if you want to make sure you have nutritious, delicious, and quality meals for you and your family, having a vegan pantry is halfway there.

Why You Ought to Reduce Your Intake of Processed and Animal-Based Foods

You have heard over and over that processed food has adverse effects on your health. You might have also been told repeatedly to stay away from foods with lots of preservatives. However, you may have never heard any genuine or concrete facts about why these foods are unsafe. Consequently, let us properly dissect it to help you properly comprehend why you ought to stay away from these offenders.

- **They have massive habit-forming characteristics**

Humans have a predisposition toward being addicted to some specific foods; however, the reality is that the fault is not wholly ours.

Every one of the unhealthy treats we relish now and then triggers a dopamine release. This creates a pleasurable effect in our brain, but the excitement is usually short-lived. The discharged dopamine gradually causes an attachment, and this is the reason some people consistently go back to eat certain unhealthy foods even when they know they're unhealthy and unnecessary. You can get rid of this by avoiding the temptation completely.

- **They are sugar-laden and heavy in glucose-fructose syrup**

Animal-based and processed foods are laden with refined sugars and glucose-fructose syrup, which has almost no nutritional value. An ever-increasing number of studies are affirming what several people presumed from the start: that genetically modified foods bring about inflammatory bowel disease, which consequently makes it increasingly difficult for the body to assimilate essential nutrients. The disadvantages that result from your body being unable to assimilate essential nutrients from consumed foods rightly cannot be overemphasized.

Processed and animal-based food products contain plenteous amounts of refined carbohydrates. Indeed, your body requires carbohydrates to give it energy to function.

In any case, refining carbs dispenses with the fundamental supplements in the way that refining entire grains disposes of the whole grain part. What remains in the wake of refining is what's considered empty carbs or empty calories. These can negatively affect the metabolic system in your body by sharply increasing your blood sugar and insulin levels.

- **They contain lots of synthetic ingredients**

When your body takes in non-natural ingredients, it regards them as a foreign substance and a health threat. It isn't accustomed to identifying synthetic compounds like sucralose or synthesized sugars. Hence, in defense of your health against this foreign "aggressor," your body does what it's programmed to do to safeguard your health: It sets off an immune reaction to tackle this "enemy" compound, which indirectly weakens your body's general disease alertness, making you susceptible to illnesses. The energy expended by your body in triggering your immune system could be better utilized somewhere else.

- **They contain constituent elements that set off a sensation in your body**

A part of processed and animal-based foods contains compounds like glucose-fructose syrup, monosodium glutamate, and specific food dyes that can trigger some addictions. They teach your body to receive a benefit whenever you consume them. Monosodium glutamate, for example, is added to many store-bought baked foods. This additive slowly conditions your palate to relish and crave the taste.

- **This reward-centric arrangement makes you crave it increasingly, which ends up exposing you to the danger of over-consuming calories**

For animal protein, usually, the expression "subpar" is used to allude to plant proteins since they generally have lower levels of essential amino acids as against animal-sourced protein. Nevertheless, what the vast majority don't know is that large amounts of essential amino acids can prove detrimental to your health. Let me break it down further for you.

- **Animal-sourced protein has no fiber**

In their pursuit to consume animal protein, the vast majority wind up dislodging the plant protein that was previously available in their body. Replacing the plant proteins with its animal variant is harmful because, in contrast to plant protein, animal proteins typically are deficient in fiber, phyto-nutrients, and antioxidant properties. Fiber insufficiency is a regular feature across various regions and societies on the planet. In America, for example, according to the National Academy of Medicine, the typical adult takes in roughly 15 grams of dietary fiber daily rather than the recommended daily quantity of 25 to 30 grams. A deficiency in dietary fiber often leads to a heightened risk of breast and colorectal cancers, in addition to constipation, inflammatory bowel disease, and cardiovascular disease.

- **Animal protein brings about an upsurge in phosphorus levels in the body**

Animal protein has significant levels of phosphorus. Our bodies stabilize these plenteous amounts of phosphorus by producing and discharging a hormone known as fibroblast growth factor 23 (FGF23). Studies have shown that this hormone is dangerous to our veins. FGF23 also causes asymmetrical expansion of heart muscles—a determinant for congestive heart failure and even mortality in some advanced cases.

Having discussed the many problems associated with animal protein, it becomes more apt to replace its "high quality" perception with the tag "highly hazardous." In contrast to caffeine, which has a withdrawal effect if it's discontinued abruptly, you can stop taking processed and animal-based foods right away without any withdrawals. Possibly the only thing that you'll give up is the ease of some meals taking little to no time to prepare.

Health Benefits of the Plant-Based Diet

Plant-based eating is one of the healthiest diets in the world. It should include plenty of fresh products, whole grains, legumes, and healthy fats such as seeds and nuts, which are rich in antioxidants, minerals, vitamins, and dietary fiber.

Scientific research has shown that higher use of plant-based foods is connected to a lower risk of death from conditions such as cardiovascular disease, diabetes, hypertension, and obesity. Vegan eating relies heavily on healthy staples, avoiding animal products. Animal products contain much more fat than plant-based foods; it's not a shocker that studies have shown that meat-eaters have nine times the obesity rate of vegans.

This leads us to the next point, one of the greatest benefits of the vegan diet: weight loss. While many people choose to live a vegan life for ethical reasons, the diet itself can help you achieve your weight loss goals. If you're struggling to shift pounds, you may want to consider trying a plant-based diet. How exactly? As a vegan, you will reduce the number of high-calorie foods such as full-fat dairy products, fatty fish, pork, and other cholesterol-containing foods such as eggs. Try replacing such foods with high-fiber and protein-rich alternatives that will keep you fuller longer. The key is focusing on nutrient-dense, clean and natural foods and avoiding empty calories such as sugar, saturated fats, and highly processed foods. Here are a few tricks that help me maintain my weight on the vegan diet. I eat vegetables as a main course; I consume good fats in moderation (good fats such as olive oil do not make you fat); I exercise regularly and cook at home. Plant foods are an excellent source of many nutrients that boost the body's metabolism in many ways. They are easy to digest thanks to their rich content of antioxidants.

- **Reduced Risk of Heart Diseases**

Processed and animal foods are responsible for much heart disease. A whole foods plant-based diet is better at nourishing the body with essential nutrients while improving the heart's function to produce and transport blood to and from the various body parts.

- **Prevents and Heals Diabetes**

Plant-based foods are excellent at reducing high blood sugar. Many studies comparing a vegetarian and vegan diet to a regular meat-filled diet proved that dieting with more plant foods reduced the risk of diabetes by 50 percent.

- **Improved Cognitive Incline**

Fruits and vegetables are excellent for cleansing and boosting metabolism. They release high numbers of plant compounds and antioxidants that slow or prevent cognitive decline. On a plant-based diet, the brain is boosted with sustainable energy, promoting sharp memory, language, thinking, and judgment abilities.

- **Quick Weight Loss**

A high animal food diet is known to drive weight gain. Switching to a plant-based diet helps the body shed fat walls easily, which quickly drives weight loss.

BREAKFAST

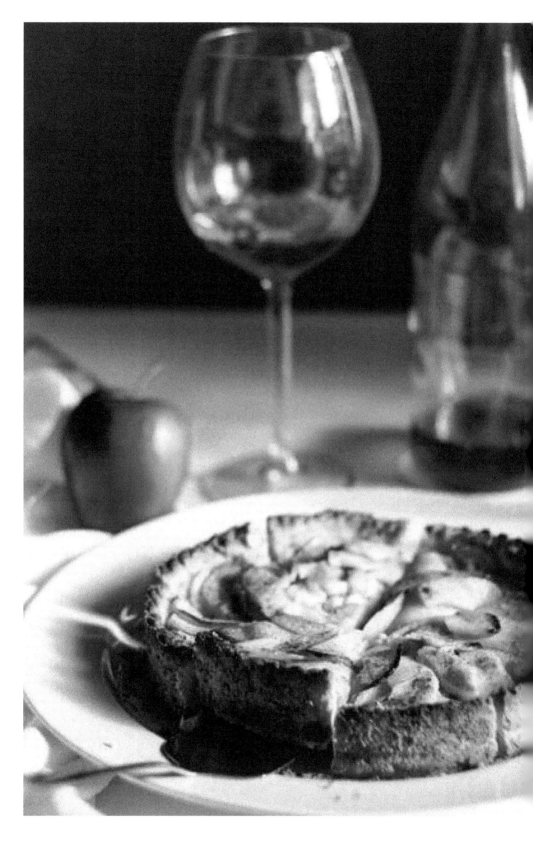

Coconut Porridge with Strawberries

4 Servings

Preparation Time: 12 minutes

Ingredients

- 2 tbsps Flax seed powder
- 2 tbsps Coconut flour
- 2 pinch Ground Chia seeds
- 5 tbsps Coconut cream
- 2 oz Olive oil
- Thawed frozen Strawberries

Directions

- In a small bowl, mix the flax seed powder with the 3 tbsps water, and allow soaking for 5 minutes.

- Put a non-stick saucepan over low heat and pour in the olive oil, vegan "flax egg," coconut flour, Chia seeds, and coconut cream.

- Cook the mixture while stirring continuously until your desired consistency is achieved.

- Turn the heat off and spoon the porridge into serving bowls.

- Top with 4 to 6 strawberries and serve immediately.

Broccoli Hash Browns

6 Servings

Preparation Time: 35 minutes

Ingredients

- 3 tbsps Flax seed powder
- ½ white onion, grated
- 1 tsp Salt
- 1 tbsp freshly ground Black pepper
- 1 head Broccoli, cut into florets
- 5 tbsps plant butter, for frying

Directions

- In a small bowl, mix the flax seed powder with 9 tbsps water, and allow soaking for 5 minutes.

- Add the broccoli into a blender and blend a few times until smoothly grated.

- Transfer the broccoli into a bowl, add the vegan "flax egg," white onion, salt, and black pepper.

- With a spoon, mix the ingredients evenly and set aside 5 to 10 minutes to firm up a bit.

- Put a large non-stick pan over medium heat and drop 1/3 of the plant butter to melt until no longer shimmering.

- Ladle scoops of the broccoli mixture into the skillet (about 3 to 4 hash browns per batch).

- Flatten the pancakes to measure 3 to 4 inches in diameter, and fry until golden brown on one side, 4 minutes.

- Turn the pancakes with a spatula and cook the other side to brown too, another 5 minutes.

- Transfer the hash browns to a serving plate and repeat the frying process for the remaining broccoli mixture.

- Serve the hash browns warm with a green salad.

No-Bread Avocado Sandwich

4 Servings

Preparation Time: 10 minutes

Ingredients

- 2 Avocados, sliced
- 4 oz gem Lettuce leaves
- 1 oz Plant butter
- 2 oz Tofu, sliced
- 2 large red tomatoes, sliced
- Freshly chopped parsley to garnish

Directions

- Put the avocado on a plate and place the tomato slices by the avocado.

- Arrange the lettuce (with the inner side facing you) on a flat plate to serve as the base of the sandwich.

- Assemble the sandwich, smear each leaf of the lettuce with plant butter, and arrange some tofu slices in the leaves.

- Share the avocado and tomato slices on each cheese. Garnish with parsley and serve.

6 Servings

Preparation Time: 46 minutes

Ingredients

- 8 oz water-packed extra firm Tofu
- 1 green Bell pepper, finely chopped
- 1 Tomato, finely chopped
- 2 tbsps freshly chopped Scallions
- Salt and Black pepper to taste
- 1 tsp Mexican-style Chili powder
- 2 tbsps Plant butter for frying
- 3 oz grated Plant-based Parmesan

Directions

- Put the tofu in between two parchment papers to drain liquid for about 30 minutes.

- Melt the plant butter in a large non-stick skillet until no longer foaming.

- Crumble the tofu into the plant butter and fry until golden brown, stirring occasionally, making sure not to break the tofu into tiny pieces.

- The goal is to have the tofu like scrambled eggs, about 4 to 6 minutes.

- Mix in the bell pepper, tomato, scallions, and cook until the vegetables are soft, about 4 minutes.

- Season with salt, black pepper, chili powder, and stir in the cheese to incorporate and melt for about 2 minutes.

- Spoon the scramble into a serving platter and serve warm.

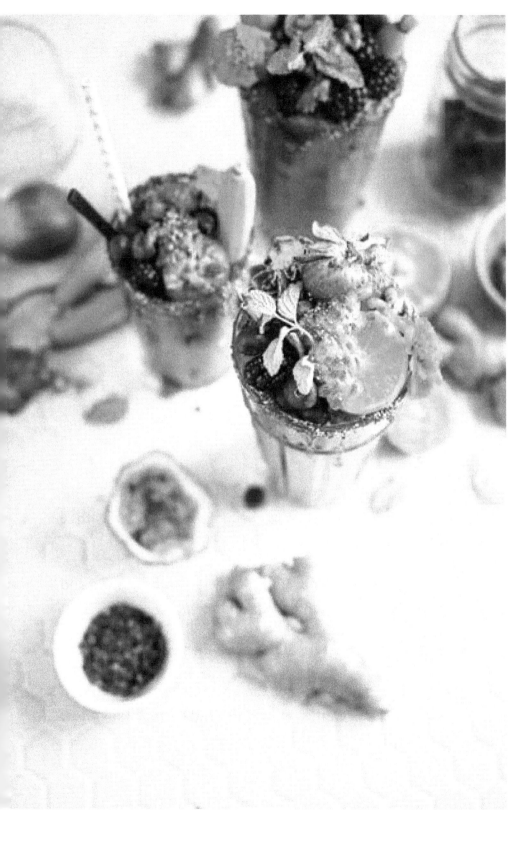

Lemon-Almond Waffles

6 Servings

Preparation Time: 20 minutes

Ingredients

- 3 tbsps Flax seed powder
- A pinch Salt
- 2 cups Almond milk
- 3 tbsps Plant butter
- 2 cups fresh Almond butter
- 2 tbsps pure Maple syrup
- 2/3 cup Almond flour
- 2 ½ tsps Baking powder
- 1 tsp fresh Lemon juice

Directions

- In a medium bowl, mix the flaxseed powder with 6 tbsps water and allow soaking for 5 minutes.

- Add in the almond flour, baking powder, salt, and almond milk. Mix until well combined.

- Preheat a waffle iron and brush with some plant butter.

- Pour in a quarter cup of the batter, close the iron and cook until the waffles are golden and crisp, 2-3 minutes.

- Transfer the waffles to a plate and make more waffles using the same process and ingredient proportions.

- In a bowl, mix the almond butter with the maple syrup and lemon juice.

- Spread the top with the almond-lemon mixture and serve.

Almond Flour English Muffins

6 Servings

Preparation Time: 20 minutes

Ingredients

- 2 tbsps Flax seed powder
- 2 tbsps Almond flour
- ½ tsp Baking powder
- 1 pinch of Salt
- 3 tbsps Plant butter

Directions

- In a small bowl, mix the flax seed with 6 tbsps water until evenly combined and leave to soak for 5 minutes.

- In another bowl, mix the almond flour, baking powder, and salt.

- Pour in the vegan "flax egg" and whisk again. Let the batter sit for 5 minutes to set.

- Melt plant butter in a frying pan and add the mixture in four dollops.

- Fry until golden brown on one side, then flip the bread with a spatula and fry further until golden brown. Serve immediately.

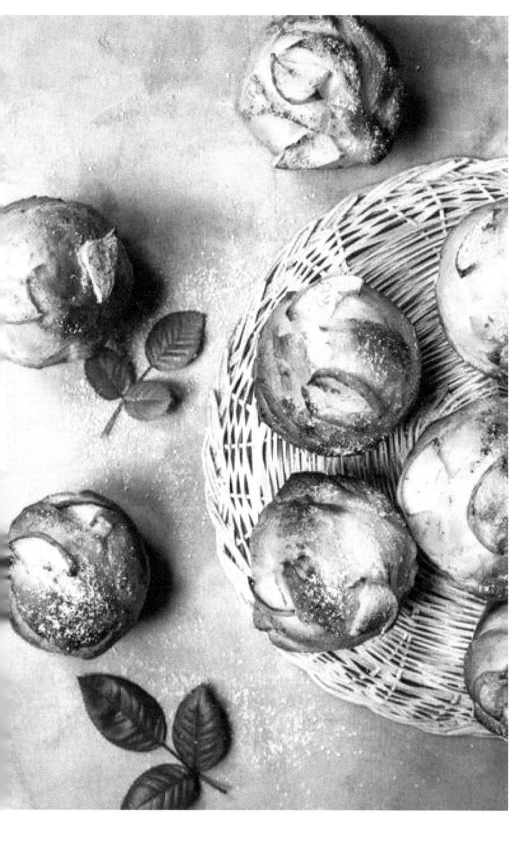

Pesto Bread Twists

8 Servings

Preparation Time: 35 minutes

Ingredients

- 1 ½ cups grated plant-based Mozzarella cheese
- ½ cup Almond flour
- ½ tsp Salt
- 1 tsp Baking powder
- 5 tbsps Plant butter
- 2 oz Pesto
- 1 tbsp Flax seed powder
- 4 tbsps Coconut flour
- Olive oil for brushing

Directions

- Mix the flax seed powder with 3 tbsps water in a bowl, and set aside to soak for 5 minutes.

- Preheat oven to 350°F and line a baking sheet with parchment paper.

- In a bowl, mix the coconut flour, almond flour, salt, and baking powder.

- Melt the plant butter and cheese in a deep pan over medium heat and stir in the vegan "flax egg." Mix in the flour mixture until a firm dough forms.

- Turn the heat off, transfer the mixture in between two parchment papers, and then use a rolling pin to flatten out the dough of about an inch's thickness.

- Remove the parchment paper on top and spread the pesto all over the dough. Now, use a knife to cut the dough into strips, twist each piece, and place it on the baking sheet.

- Brush with olive oil and bake for 15 to 20 minutes until golden brown.

- Remove the bread twist; allow cooling for a few minutes, and serve with warm almond milk.

DRINKS

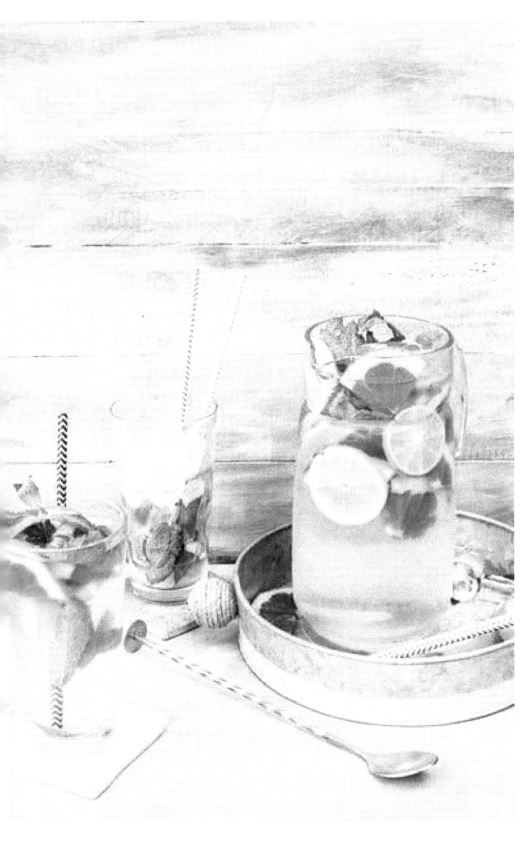

Energizing Cinnamon Detox Tonic

2 Servings

Preparation Time: 45 minutes

Ingredients

- 4 sticks of cinnamon 2 inches each
- 1 small lemon slice
- 1/8 teaspoon of cayenne pepper
- 1/8 teaspoon of ground turmeric
- 1 teaspoon of maple syrup
- 1 teaspoon of apple cider vinegar
- 2 cups of boiling water

Directions

- Pour the boiling water into a small saucepan, add and stir the cinnamon sticks, then let it rest for 8 to 10 minutes before covering the pan.
- Pass the mixture through a strainer and into the liquid; add the cayenne pepper, turmeric, cinnamon and stir properly.
- Add the maple syrup, vinegar, and lemon slice.
- Add and stir an infused lemon and serve immediately.

Warm Pomegranate Punch

12 Servings

Preparation Time: 2 hours and 15 minutes

Ingredients

- 3 cinnamon sticks, each about 3 inches long
- 12 whole cloves
- 1/2 cup of coconut sugar
- 1/3 cup of lemon juice
- 32 fluid ounces of pomegranate juice
- 32 fluid ounces of apple juice, unsweetened
- 16 fluid ounces of brewed tea

Directions

- Using a 4-quart slow cooker, pour the lemon juice, pomegranate juice, apple juice, tea, and then sugar.
- Wrap the whole cloves and cinnamon stick in cheesecloth, tie its corners with a string, and immerse it in the liquid present in the slow cooker.
- Then cover it with the lid, plug in the slow cooker and let it cook at the low heat setting for 3 hours or until it is heated thoroughly.
- When done, discard the cheesecloth bag and serve it hot or cold.

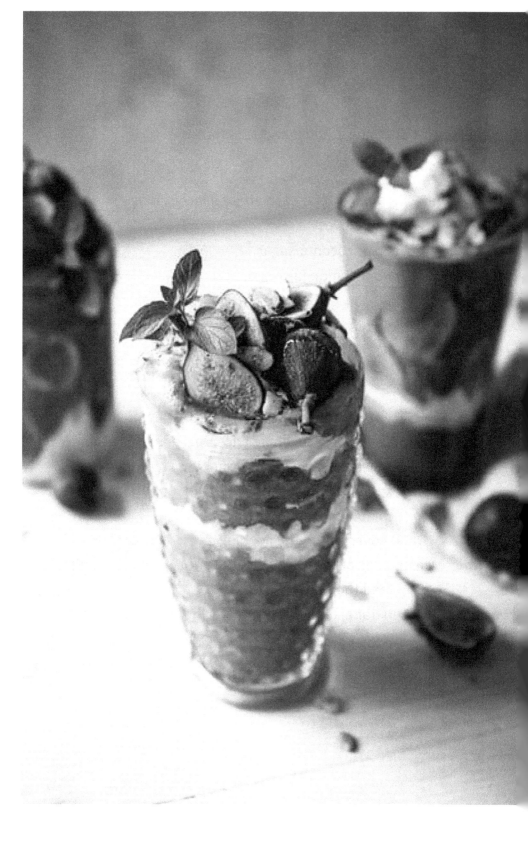

Rich Truffle Hot Chocolate

4 Servings

Preparation Time: 1 hour and 40 minutes

Ingredients

- 1/3 cup of cocoa powder, unsweetened
- 1/3 cup of coconut sugar
- 1/8 teaspoon of salt
- 1/8 teaspoon of ground cinnamon
- 1 teaspoon of vanilla extract, unsweetened
- 32 fluid ounce of coconut milk

Directions

- Using a 2 quarts slow cooker, add all the ingredients, and stir properly.
- Cover it with the lid, then plug in the slow cooker and cook it for 2 hours on the high heat setting or until it is heated thoroughly.
- When done, serve right away.

Warm Spiced Lemon Drink

12 Servings

Preparation Time: 2 hours and 40 minutes

Ingredients

- 1 cinnamon stick, about 3 inches long
- 1/2 teaspoon of whole cloves
- 2 cups of coconut sugar
- 4 fluid of ounce pineapple juice
- 1/2 cup and 2 tablespoons of lemon juice
- 12 fluid ounces of orange juice
- 2 1/2 quarts of water

Directions

- Pour water into a 6-quarts slow cooker and stir the sugar and lemon juice properly.
- Wrap the cinnamon, the whole cloves in cheesecloth, and tie its corners with string.
- Immerse this cheesecloth bag in the liquid present in the slow cooker and cover it with the lid.
- Then plug in the slow cooker and let it cook on a high heat setting for 2 hours or until it is heated thoroughly.
- When done, discard the cheesecloth bag and serve the drink hot or cold.

Ultimate Mulled Wine

6 Servings

Preparation Time: 45 minutes

Ingredients

- 1 cup of cranberries, fresh
- 2 oranges, juiced
- 1 tablespoon of whole cloves
- 2 cinnamon sticks, each about 3 inches long
- 1 tablespoon of star anise
- 1/3 cup of honey
- 8 fluid ounces of apple cider
- 8 fluid ounces of cranberry juice
- 24 fluid ounces of red wine

Directions

- Using a 4 quarts slow cooker, add all the ingredients, and stir properly.
- Cover it with the lid, then plug in the slow cooker and cook it for 30 minutes on the high heat setting or until it gets warm thoroughly.
- When done, strain the wine and serve right away.

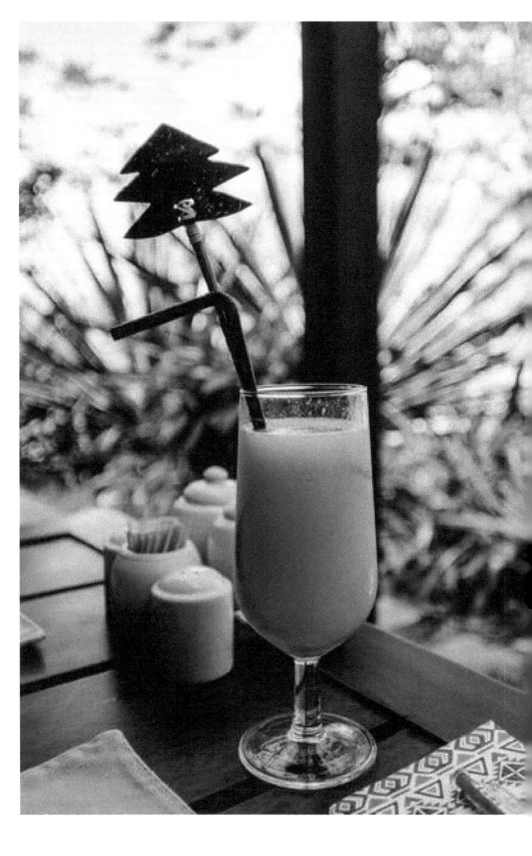

Pleasant Lemonade

6 Servings

Preparation Time: 3 hours and 45 minutes

Ingredients

- Cinnamon sticks for serving
- 2 cups of coconut sugar
- 1/4 cup of honey
- 3 cups of lemon juice. fresh
- 32 fluid ounce of water

Directions

- Using a 4-quarts slow cooker, place all the ingredients except for the cinnamon sticks and stir properly.
- Cover it with the lid, then plug in the slow cooker and cook it for 3 hours on the low heat setting or until it is heated thoroughly.
- When done, stir properly and serve with the cinnamon sticks.

LUNCH

Tofu Cabbage Stir-Fry

6 Servings

Preparation Time: 45 minutes

Ingredients

- 2 ½ cups Baby bok choy, quartered
- 2 Garlic cloves, minced
- 1 tsp Chili flakes
- 1 tbsp fresh ginger, grated
- 3 green onions, sliced
- 1 tbsp Sesame oil
- 1 cup Tofu mayonnaise
- 5 oz plant Butter
- 2 cups tofu, cubed
- 1 tsp Garlic powder
- 1 tsp Onion powder
- 1 tbsp plain Vinegar

Directions

- Melt half of the butter in a wok over medium heat, add the bok choy, and stir-fry until softened. Season with salt, black pepper, garlic powder, onion powder, and plain vinegar. Sauté for 2 minutes; set aside.

- Melt the remaining butter in the wok, add and sauté garlic, chili flakes, and ginger until fragrant.

- Put the tofu in the wok and cook until browned on all sides.

- Add the green onions and bok choy, heat for 2 minutes, and add the sesame oil.

- Stir in tofu mayonnaise, cook for 2 minutes, and serve.

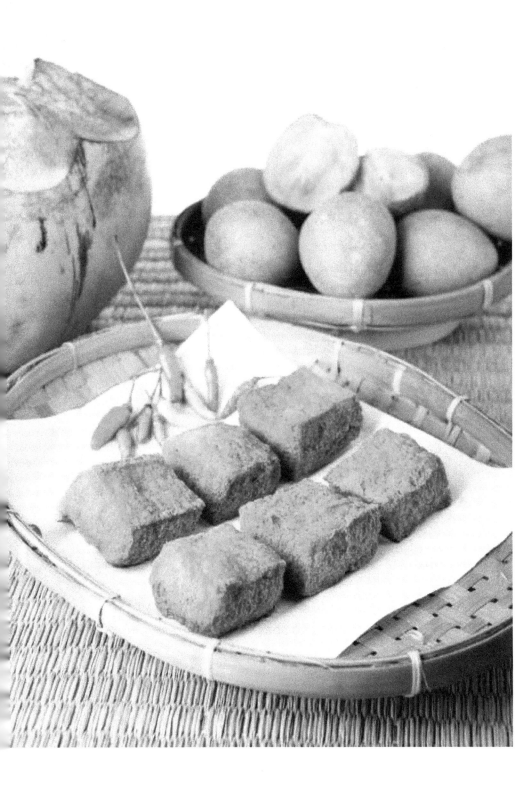

Smoked Tempeh with Broccoli Fritters

5 Servings

Preparation Time: 40 minutes

Ingredients

- 4 tbsps Flax seed powder
- 1 tbsp Soy sauce
- 8 oz Tofu, grated
- 3 tbsps Almond flour
- ½ tsp Onion powder
- 4 ¼ oz plant butter
- ½ cup mixed Salad greens
- 1 cup tofu Mayonnaise
- Juice of ½ a Lemon
- 3 tbsps Olive oil
- 1 tbsp grated Ginger
- 3 tbsps fresh Lime juice
- Cayenne pepper to taste
- 10 oz Tempeh slices
- 1 head Broccoli, grated

Directions

- Take a bowl, mix the flax seed powder with 12 tbsps water and set aside to soak for 5 minutes.

- In another bowl, combine soy sauce, olive oil, grated ginger, lime juice, salt, and cayenne pepper.

- Brush the tempeh slices with the mixture.

- Heat a grill pan over medium and grill the tempeh on both sides until golden brown and nicely smoked. Remove the slices to a plate.

- In another bowl, mix the tofu with broccoli.

- Add in vegan "flax egg," almond flour, onion powder, salt, and black pepper. Mix and form 12 patties out of the mixture.

- Melt the plant butter in a pan and fry the patties on both sides until golden brown. Remove to a plate.

- Add the grilled tempeh with the broccoli fritters and salad greens.

- Mix the tofu mayonnaise with the lemon juice and drizzle over the salad.

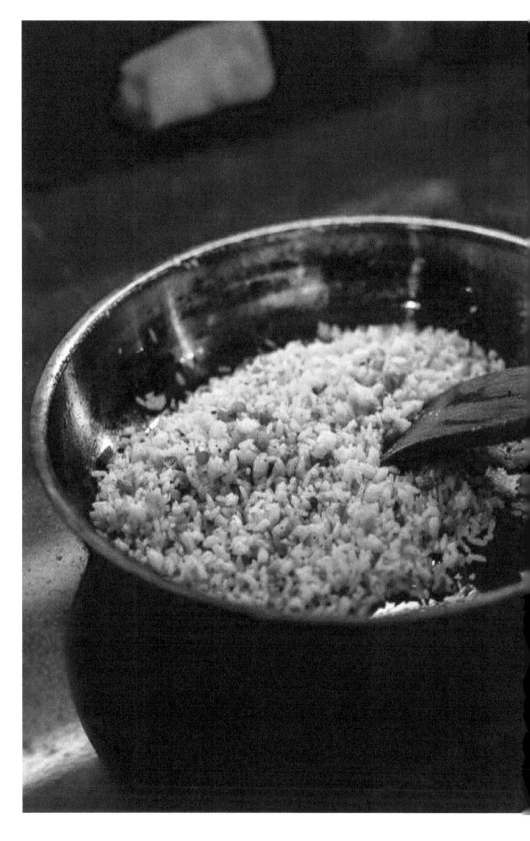

Spicy Veggie Steaks with Green Salad

6 Servings

Preparation Time: 35 minutes

Ingredients

- 1 Eggplant, sliced
- 1 oz mixed Salad greens
- ½ cup tofu Mayonnaise
- Salt to taste
- ½ tsp Cayenne pepper to taste
- 1 Zucchini, sliced
- ¼ cup Coconut oil
- Juice of ½ a Lemon
- 5 oz plant-based Cheddar, cubed
- 10 Kalamata Olives
- 2 tbsps Pecans

Directions

- Set oven to broil and line a baking sheet with parchment paper.

- Arrange eggplant and zucchini on the baking sheet.

- Brush with coconut oil and sprinkle with cayenne pepper. Broil for 15-20 minutes.

- Remove to a serving platter and drizzle with the lemon juice.

- Arrange the plant-based cheddar cheese, Kalamata olives, pecans, and mixed greens with the grilled veggies.

- Top with tofu mayonnaise and serve.

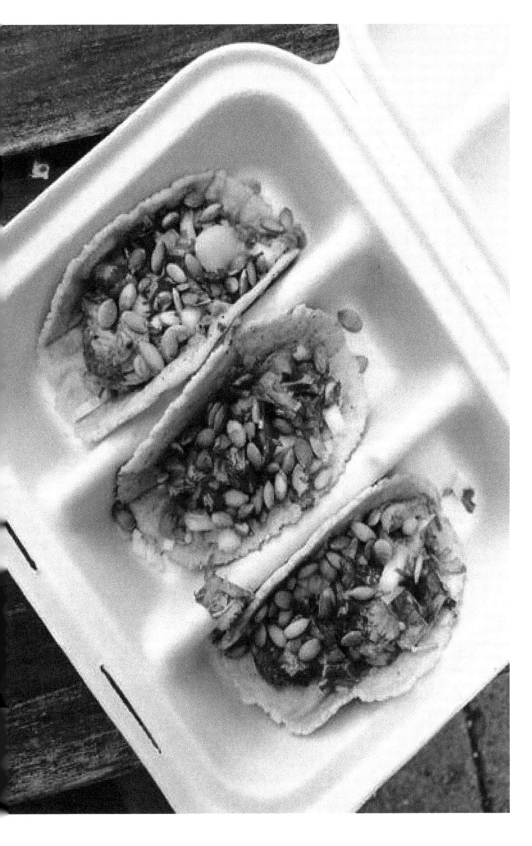

Mushroom Curry Pie

4 Servings

Preparation Time: 70 minutes

Ingredients

Piecrust

- 1 tbsp flax Seed powder + 3 tbsps water
- ¾ cup Coconut flour
- 4 tbsps Chia seeds
- 4 tbsps Almond flour
- 1 tbsp Psyllium husk powder
- 1 tsp Baking powder
- 1 pinch of Salt
- 3 tbsps Olive oil
- 4 tbsps Water

Filling

- 1 cup chopped shiitake mushrooms
- 1 cup tofu Mayonnaise
- ½ tsp Paprika
- ½ tsp Garlic powder
- ½ cup Cashew cream cheese
- 1 ¼ cups grated Plant-based Parmesan
- 3 tbsps Flax seed powder + 9 tbsps water
- ½ red Bell pepper, finely chopped
- 1 tsp Turmeric

Directions

- In two separate bowls, mix the different portions of flax seed powder with the respective quantity of water and set aside to absorb for 5 minutes.

- Preheat oven to 350 F.

- When the vegan "flax egg" is ready, pour the smaller quantity into a food processor, add in the pie crust ingredients and blend until a ball forms out of the dough.

- Line a spring-form pan with parchment paper and grease with cooking spray.

- Spread the dough on the bottom of the pan and bake for 15 minutes.

- In a bowl, add the remaining flax egg and all the filling ingredients, combine the mixture, and fill the piecrust. Bake for 40 minutes. Serve sliced.

Tofu & Spinach Lasagna with Red Sauce

5 Servings

Preparation Time: 65 minutes

Ingredients

- 2 tbsps Plant butter
- 1 white Onion, chopped
- 1 garlic Clove, minced
- 2 ½ cups Crumbled tofu
- 3 tbsps Tomato paste
- ½ tbsp Dried oregano
- Salt and Black pepper to taste
- 5 oz grated plant-based mozzarella
- 2 oz grated plant-based Parmesan
- ½ cup fresh parsley, finely chopped
- 1 cup Baby Spinach
- 8 tbsps Flax seed powder
- 1 ½ cups Cashew cream cheese
- 5 tbsps Psyllium husk powder
- 2 cups Coconut cream

Directions

- Melt plant butter in a medium pot and sauté onion and garlic until fragrant and soft, about 3 minutes.

- Stir in tofu and cook until brown.

- Mix in tomato paste, oregano, salt, and black pepper.

- Pour ½ cup of water into the pot, stir, and simmer the ingredients until most of the liquid has evaporated.

- Preheat oven to 300 F.

- Mix flax seed powder with 1 ½ cups water in a bowl to make vegan "flax egg." Allow sitting to thicken for 5 minutes.

- Combine vegan "flax egg" with cashew cream cheese and salt.

- Add psyllium husk powder a bit at a time while whisking and allow the mixture to sit for a few minutes.

- Line a baking sheet with parchment paper and spread the mixture in. Cover with another parchment paper and flatten the dough into the sheet.

- Bake for 10-12 minutes. Slice the pasta into sheets.

- In a bowl, combine coconut cream and two-thirds of the plant-based mozzarella cheese.

- Fetch out 2 tablespoons of the mixture and reserve.

- Combine in plant-based Parmesan cheese, salt, pepper, and parsley. Set aside.

- Grease a baking dish with cooking spray, layer a single line of pasta, spread with some tomato sauce, 1/3 of the spinach, and ¼ of the coconut cream mixture.

- Repeat layering the ingredients twice in the same manner, making sure to top the final layer with the coconut cream mixture and the reserved cream cheese.

- Bake for 30 minutes at 400 F.

- Slice and serve with salad.

Curried Tofu with Buttery Cabbage
6 Servings

Preparation Time: 55 minutes

Ingredients

- 2 cups tofu, cubed
- 1 tbsp + 3 ½ tbsp Coconut oil
- ½ cup grated Coconut
- 4 oz plant Butter
- Salt and Black pepper to taste
- Lemon wedges for serving
- 1 tsp yellow Curry powder
- ½ tsp Onion powder
- 2 cups Napa Cabbage, grated

Directions

- Drizzle 1 tablespoon of coconut oil on the tofu.

- In a bowl, mix the shredded coconut, yellow curry powder, salt, and onion powder.

- Toss the tofu cubes in the spice mixture.

- Heat the remaining coconut oil in a non-stick skillet and fry the coated tofu until golden brown on all sides. Transfer to a plate.

- In another skillet, melt half of the plant butter, add, and sauté the cabbage until slightly caramelized.

- Then, season with salt and black pepper.

- Dish the cabbage into serving plates with tofu and lemon wedges.

- Melt the remaining plant butter in the skillet and drizzle over the cabbage and tofu. Serve it.

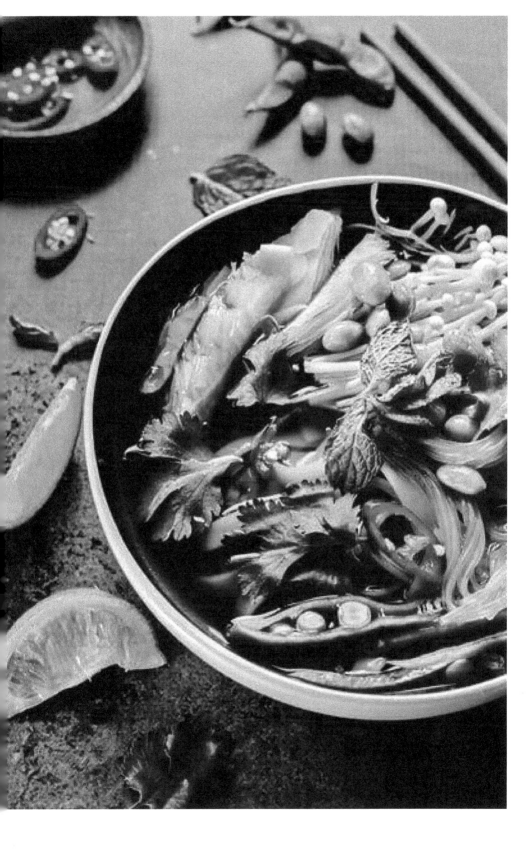

Avocado Coconut Pie

6 Servings

Preparation Time: 80 minutes

Ingredients

Piecrust

- 1 tbsp Flax seed powder + 3 tbsps water
- 1 cup Coconut flour
- 1 tsp Baking soda
- 1 pinch Salt
- 3 tbsps Coconut oil
- 4 tbsps Water
- 4 tbsps Chia seeds
- 1 tbsp Psyllium husk powder

Filling

- 2 ripe Avocados, chopped
- ½ tsp Onion powder
- ¼ tsp Salt
- ½ cup Cream cheese
- 1 ¼ cups grated Plant-based Parmesan
- 1 cup Tofu mayonnaise
- 3 tbsps flax Seed powder + 9 tbsps water
- 2 tbsps fresh Parsley, chopped
- 1 Jalapeno, finely chopped

Directions

- In 2 separate bowls, mix the different portions of flax seed powder with the respective quantity of water. Allow absorbing for 5 minutes.

- Preheat oven to 350 F.

- In a food processor, add the piecrust ingredients and the smaller portion of the vegan "flax egg."

- Mix until the resulting dough forms into a ball.

- Line a spring form pan with parchment paper and spread the dough in the pan.

- Bake for 10-15 minutes.

- Add the avocado in a bowl and add the tofu mayonnaise, remaining vegan "flax egg," parsley, jalapeno, onion powder, salt, cream cheese, and plant-based Parmesan. Combine well.

- Remove the piecrust when ready and fill with the creamy mixture. Bake for 35 minutes. Cool before slicing and serving.

Green Avocado Carbonara

6 Servings

Preparation Time: 30 minutes

Ingredients

- 8 tbsps flax seed powder
- 1 ½ cups cashew cream cheese
- 5 ½ tbsps psyllium husk powder
- 1 avocado, chopped
- 1 ¾ cups coconut cream
- Juice of ½ lemon
- 1 teaspoon onion powder
- ½ teaspoon garlic powder
- ¼ cup olive oil
- Salt and black pepper to taste
- ½ cup grated plant-based Parmesan
- 4 tbsps toasted pecans

Directions

- Preheat oven to 300 F.

- In a medium bowl, mix the flax seed powder with 1 ½ cups water and allow sitting to thicken for 5 minutes.

- Add the cashew cream cheese, salt, and psyllium husk powder.

- Whisk until smooth batter forms. Line a baking sheet with parchment paper, pour in the batter, and cover with another parchment paper.

- Use a rolling pin to flatten the dough into the sheet. Bake for 10-12 minutes. Remove, take off the parchment papers and use a sharp knife to slice the pasta into thin strips lengthwise.

- Cut each piece into halves, pour into a bowl, and set aside.

- In a blender, combine avocado, coconut cream, lemon juice, onion powder, and garlic powder; puree until smooth.

- Pour the olive oil over the pasta and stir to coat properly. Pour the avocado sauce on top and mix.

- Season with salt and black pepper.

- Divide the pasta into serving plates, garnish with Parmesan cheese and pecans, and serve immediately.

SNACKS & SIDES

12 Servings

Preparation time: 35 minutes

Ingredients

- 1 cup unsweetened almond milk
- ½ cup coconut flour
- ½ tsp cayenne pepper
- 1 cup whole-grain breadcrumbs
- 1 cup grated plant-based mozzarella
- 50 oz cauliflower florets
- 2 lb parsnips, peeled and quartered
- 6 tbsps melted plant butter
- A pinch of nutmeg
- 2 tsps cumin powder
- 2 cups coconut cream
- 4 tbsps sesame oil

Directions

- Preheat oven to 425 F and line a baking sheet with parchment paper.

- In a small bowl, combine almond milk, coconut flour, and cayenne pepper.

- In another bowl, mix salt, breadcrumbs, and plant-based mozzarella cheese.

- Dip each cauliflower floret into the milk mixture, coating properly, and then into the cheese mixture.

- Place the breaded cauliflower on the baking sheet and bake in the oven for 30 minutes, turning once after 15 minutes.

- Make slightly salted water in a saucepan and add the parsnips.

- Bring to boil over medium heat for 15 minutes or until the parsnips are fork-tender. Drain and transfer to a bowl.

- Add in melted plant butter, cumin powder, nutmeg, and coconut cream.

- Puree the ingredients using an immersion blender until smooth.

- Spoon the parsnip mash into serving plates and drizzle with some sesame oil.

- Serve with the baked cauliflower when ready.

Spinach Chips with Guacamole Hummus

8 Servings

Preparation time: 30 minutes

Ingredients

- 1 cup baby spinach
- 2 tbsps olive oil
- 1 tsp plain vinegar
- 6 large avocados, chopped
- 1 cup chopped parsley + for garnish
- 1 cup melted plant butter
- ½ cup pumpkin seeds
- ½ cup sesame paste
- Juice from 1 lemon
- 2 garlic clove, minced
- 1 tsp coriander powder
- Salt and black pepper to taste

Directions

- Preheat oven to 300 F.

- Put spinach in a bowl and toss with olive oil, vinegar, and salt.

- Place in a parchment paper-lined baking sheet and bake until the leaves are crispy but not burned, about 15 minutes.

- Place avocado into the bowl of a food processor.

- Add in parsley, plant butter, pumpkin seeds, sesame paste, lemon juice, garlic, coriander powder, salt, and black pepper.

- Puree until smooth.

- Spoon the hummus into a bowl and garnish with parsley. Serve with spinach chips.

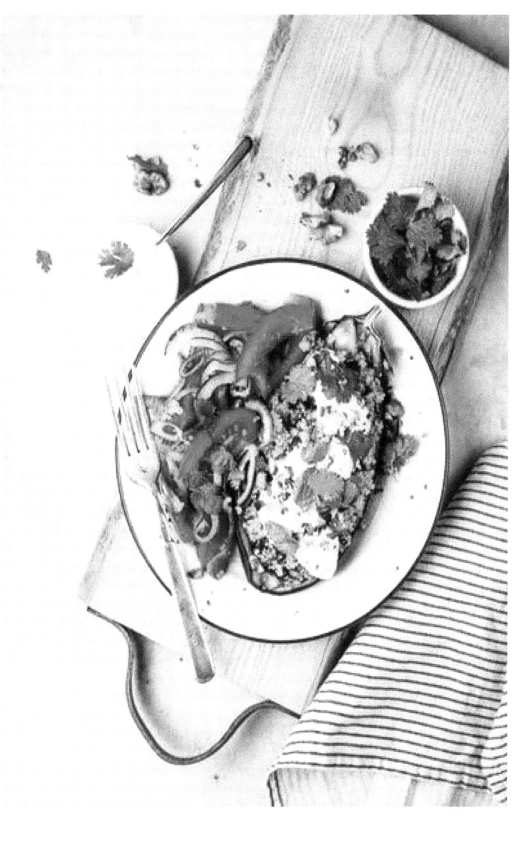

Buttered Carrot Noodles with Kale

8 Servings

Preparation time: 15 minutes

Ingredients

- 4 large carrots
- ½ cup vegetable broth
- 8 tbsps plant butter
- 2 garlic clove, minced
- 2 cups chopped kale
- Salt and black pepper to taste

Directions

- Peel the carrots with a slicer and run both through a spiralizer to form noodles.

- Pour the vegetable broth into a saucepan and add the carrot noodles.

- Simmer (over low heat) the carrots for 3 minutes.

- Strain through a colander and set the vegetables aside.

- Place a large skillet over medium heat and melt the plant butter.

- Add the garlic and sauté until softened and put in the kale; cook until wilted.

- Pour the carrots into the pan, season with salt and black pepper, and stir-fry for 3 to 4 minutes.

- Spoon the vegetables into a bowl and serve with pan-grilled tofu.

Curry Cauli Rice with Mushrooms

8 Servings

Preparation time: 15 minutes

Ingredients

- 16 oz baby Bella mushrooms, stemmed and sliced
- 4 large heads of cauliflower
- 4 tbsps toasted sesame oil, divided
- 2 onions, chopped
- 6 garlic cloves, minced
- Salt and black pepper to taste
- 1 tsp curry powder
- 2 tsps freshly chopped parsley
- 4 scallions, thinly sliced

Directions

- Use a knife to cut the entire cauliflower head into 6 pieces and transfer to a food processor.

- With the grater attachment, shred the cauliflower into a rice-like consistency.

- Heat half of the sesame oil in a large skillet over medium heat, and then add the onion and mushrooms.

- Sauté for 5 minutes or until the mushrooms are soft.

- Add the garlic and sauté for 2 minutes or until fragrant.

- Pour in the cauliflower and cook until the rice has slightly softened for about 10 minutes.

- Season with salt, black pepper, and curry powder; then, mix the ingredients to be well combined.

- After, turn the heat off and stir in the parsley and scallions.

- Dish the cauli rice into serving plates and serve warm.

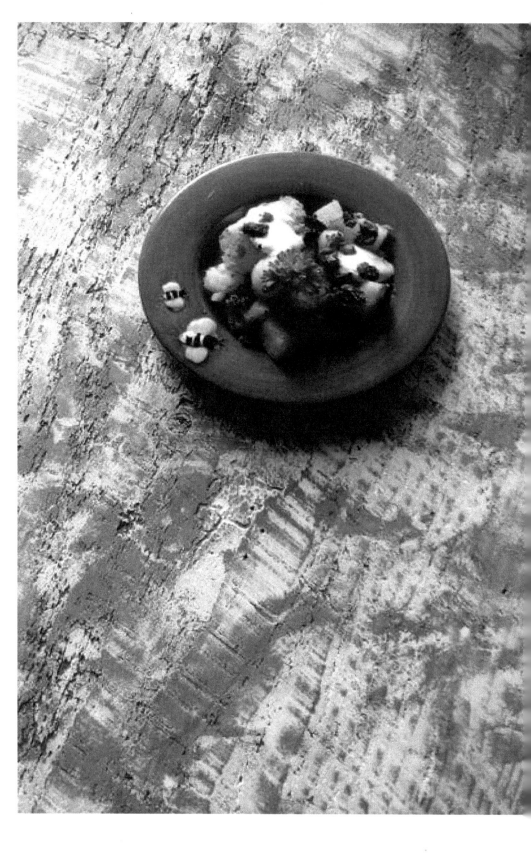

Mixed Seed Crackers

6 Servings

Preparation time: 57 minute

Ingredients

- 2/3 cup sesame seed flour
- 2/3 cup pumpkin seeds
- 2/3 cup sunflower seeds
- 2/3 cup sesame seeds
- 2/3 cup Chia seeds
- 2 tbsps psyllium husk powder
- 2 tsps salt
- ½ cup plant butter, melted
- 2 cups boiling water

Directions

- Preheat oven to 300 F.

- Combine the sesame seed flour with the pumpkin seeds, sunflower seeds, sesame seeds, Chia seeds, psyllium husk powder, and salt.

- Pour in the plant butter and hot water and mix the ingredients until a dough forms with a gel-like consistency.

- Line a baking sheet with parchment paper and place the dough on the sheet.

- Cover the dough with another parchment paper and, with a rolling pin, flatten the dough into the baking sheet.

- Remove the parchment paper on top.

- Tuck the baking sheet in the oven and bake for 45 minutes.

- Allow the crackers to cool and dry in the oven, about 10 minutes.

- After, remove the sheet and break the crackers into small pieces. Serve.

Mushroom Broccoli Faux Risotto

8 Servings

Preparation time: 25 minutes

Ingredients

- 8 oz plant butter
- 2 cups cremini mushrooms, chopped
- 4 garlic cloves, minced
- 2 small red onions, finely chopped
- 2 large head broccolis, grated
- 1 ½ cups white wine
- 2 cups coconut whipping cream
- 1 ½ cups grated plant-based Parmesan
- Freshly chopped thyme

Directions

- Place a pot over medium heat, add, and melt the plant butter.

- Sauté the mushrooms in the pot until golden, about 5 minutes.

- Add the garlic and onions and cook for 3 minutes or until fragrant and soft.

- Mix in the broccoli, 1 cup water, and half of the white wine.

- Season with salt and black pepper and simmer the ingredients (uncovered) for 8 to 10 minutes or until the broccoli are soft.

- Mix in the coconut whipping cream and simmer until most of the cream has evaporated.

- Turn the heat off and stir in the parmesan cheese and thyme until well incorporated.

- Dish the risotto and serve warm as itself or with grilled tofu.

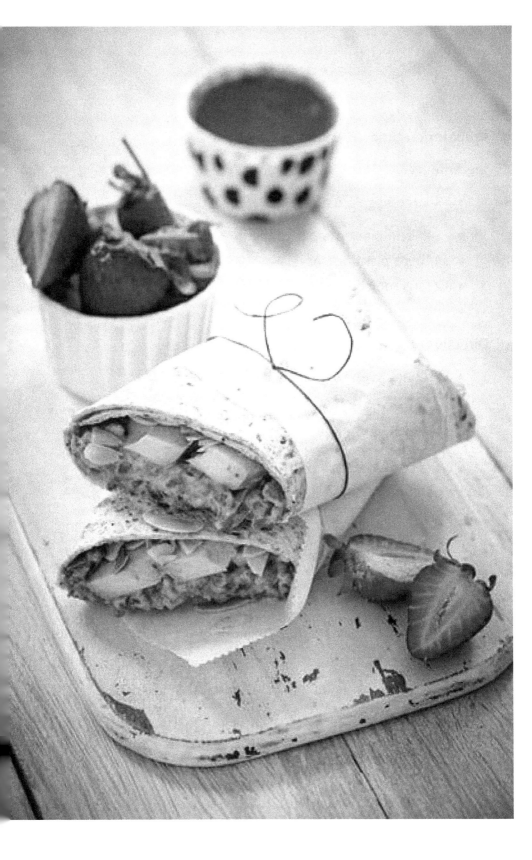

Baked Spicy Eggplant

8 Servings

Preparation time: 30 minutes

Ingredients

- 4 large eggplants

- Salt and black pepper to taste
- 4 tbsps plant butter
- 2 tsps red chili flakes
- 8 oz raw ground almonds

Directions

- Preheat oven to 400 F.

- Cut off the head of the eggplants and slice the body into 2-inch rounds.

- Season with salt and black pepper and arrange on a parchment paper-lined baking sheet.

- Drop thin slices of the plant butter on each eggplant slice, sprinkle with red chili flakes, and bake in the oven for 20 minutes.

- Slide the baking sheet out and sprinkle with the almonds. Roast further for 5 minutes or until golden brown.

- Dish the eggplants and serve with arugula salad.

SOUPS & SALADS

Spinach & Kale Soup with Fried Collards

6 Servings

Preparation Time: 16 minutes

Ingredients

- 4 tbsps Plant butter
- 3 tbsps chopped Fresh mint leaves
- Salt and Black pepper to taste
- Juice from 1 Lime
- 1 cup Collard greens, chopped
- 2 Garlic cloves, minced
- 1 pinch of green Cardamom powder
- 1 cup fresh spinach, chopped
- 1 cup fresh kale, chopped
- 1 large Avocado
- 3 ½ cups Coconut cream
- 4 cups Vegetable broth

Directions

- Melt 2 tbsps of plant butter in a saucepan over medium heat and sauté spinach and kale for 5 minutes.

- Turn the heat off. Add in the avocado, coconut cream, vegetable broth, salt, and pepper.

- Puree the ingredients with an immersion blender until smooth. Pour in the lime juice and set aside.

- Melt the remaining plant butter in a pan and add the collard greens, garlic, and cardamom; sauté until the garlic is fragrant and has achieved a golden brown color, about 4 minutes.

- Fetch the soup into serving bowls and garnish with fried collards and mint. Serve warm.

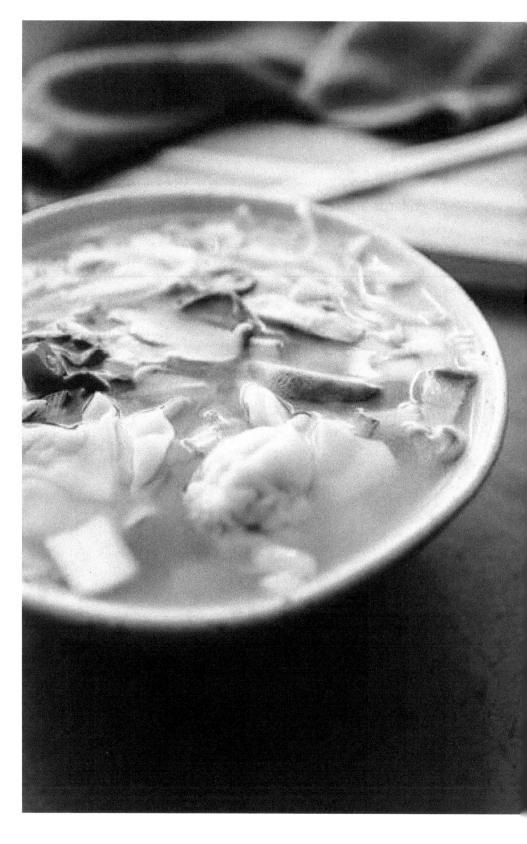

Tofu Goulash Soup

6 Servings

Preparation Time: 25 minutes

Ingredients

- 1 ½ cups extra-firm tofu, crumbled
- 1 tbsp dried basil
- ½ tbsp crushed Cardamom seeds
- Salt and Black pepper to taste
- 1 ½ cups crushed Tomatoes
- 4 cups Vegetable broth
- 1 ½ tsps Red wine vinegar
- Chopped Cilantro to serve
- 3 tbsps Plant butter
- 1 white Onion
- 2 Garlic cloves
- 8 oz chopped Butternut squash
- 1 red Bell pepper
- 1 tbsp Paprika powder
- ¼ tsp Red chili flakes

Directions

- Melt plant butter in a pot over medium heat and sauté onion and garlic for 3 minutes.

- Stir in tofu and cook for 3 minutes; add the butternut squash, bell pepper, paprika, red chili flakes, basil, cardamom seeds, salt, and pepper. Cook for 2 minutes.

- Add in tomatoes and vegetable broth. Bring to a boil, reduce the heat and simmer for 10 minutes. Mix in red wine vinegar.

- Garnish with cilantro and serve.

Celery & Potato Soup

8 Servings

Preparation Time: 55 minutes

Ingredients

- 2 tbsps Olive oil
- 1 golden Beet, peeled and diced
- 1 yellow Bell pepper, chopped
- 1 Yukon Gold potato, diced
- 6 cups Vegetable broth
- 1 tsp Dried thyme
- Salt and Black pepper to taste
- 1 tbsp Lemon juice
- 1 Onion, chopped
- 1 Carrot, chopped
- 1 Celery stalk, chopped
- 2 Garlic cloves, minced

Directions

- Heat the oil in a pot over medium heat.

- Add the onion, carrot, celery, and garlic. Cook for 5 minutes or until softened.

- Stir in beet, bell pepper, and potato, cook uncovered for 1 minute.

- Pour in the broth and thyme. Season with salt and pepper.

- Cook for 45 minutes until the vegetables are tender. Serve sprinkled with lemon juice.

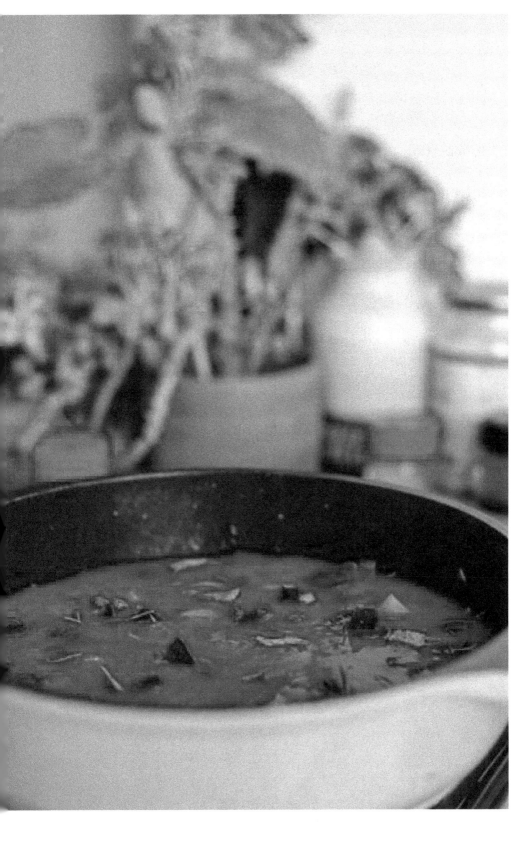

Medley of Mushroom Soup

4 Servings

Preparation Time: 40 minutes

Ingredients

- 4 oz Unsalted plant butter
- 5 oz Shiitake mushrooms, chopped
- ½ lb Celery root, chopped
- ½ tsp Dried rosemary
- 1 Vegetable stock cube, crushed
- 1 tbsp Plain vinegar
- 1 cup Coconut cream
- 4 – 6 Leaves basil, chopped
- 1 small Onion, finely chopped
- 1 clove Garlic, minced
- 5 oz button Mushrooms, chopped
- 5 oz cremini Mushrooms, chopped

Directions

- Put a saucepan over medium-high heat, add the plant butter to melt, then sauté the onion, garlic, mushrooms, and celery root in the butter until golden brown and fragrant, about 6 minutes.

- Fetch out some mushrooms and reserve for garnishing. Add the rosemary, 3 cups of water, stock cube, and vinegar.

- Stir the mixture and bring it to a boil for 6 minutes. After, reduce the heat and simmer the soup for 15 minutes or until the celery is soft.

- Mix in the coconut cream and puree the ingredients using an immersion blender. Simmer for 2 minutes.

- Spoon the soup into serving bowls, garnish with the reserved mushrooms and basil. Serve.

Cauliflower Dill Soup

6 Servings

Preparation Time: 26 minutes

Ingredients

- 2 tbsps Coconut oil
- 1 tsp Cumin powder
- ¼ tsp Nutmeg powder
- 1 head Cauliflower, cut into florets
- 3 ½ cups Seasoned vegetable stock
- 5 oz Plant butter
- Juice from 1 Lemon
- ¼ cup Coconut whipping cream
- ½ lb Celery root, trimmed
- 1 Garlic clove
- 1 medium White onion
- ¼ cup Fresh dill, roughly chopped

Directions

- Place a pot over medium heat, add the coconut oil and allow heating until no longer shimmering.

- Add in the celery root, garlic clove, and onion; sauté the vegetables until fragrant and soft, about 5 minutes.

- Stir in the dill, cumin, and nutmeg, and fry further for 1 minute.

- Mix in the cauliflower florets and vegetable stock.

- Bring the soup to a boil for 12 to 15 minutes or until the cauliflower is soft. Turn the heat off.

- Add in the plant butter and lemon juice. Puree the ingredients with an immersion blender until smooth.

- Mix in coconut whipping cream and season the soup with salt and black pepper. Serve warm.

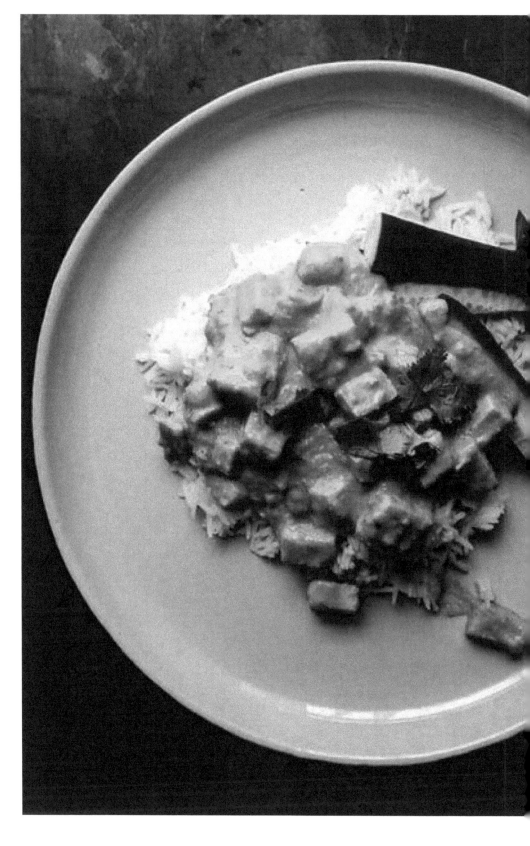

Radish & Cabbage Ginger Salad

6 Servings

Preparation Time: 15 minutes

Ingredients

- 8 oz Napa cabbage, cut crosswise into strips
- 2 tbsps Tice vinegar
- 2 tsps toasted sesame oil
- 1 tbsp Soy sauce
- 1 tsp grated Fresh ginger
- ½ tsp Dry mustard
- Salt and Black pepper to taste
- 2 tbsps chopped Roasted hazelnuts
- 1 cup grated carrots
- 1 cup sliced Radishes
- 2 green Onions, minced
- 2 tbsps chopped fresh Parsley

Directions

- Put the Napa cabbage, carrot, radishes, green onions, and parsley in a bowl, stir to combine.
- In another bowl, mix vinegar, sesame oil, soy sauce, ginger, mustard, salt, and pepper.
- Pour over the slaw and toss to coat.
- Marinate covered in the fridge for 2 hours.
- Serve topped with hazelnuts.

Lemon Potato Salad with Kalamata Olives

4 Servings

Preparation time: 30 minutes

Ingredients

- 1 tsp Dried dill
- ½ cucumber, chopped
- ¼ Red onion, diced
- ¼ cup chopped Kalamata olives
- ¼ cup chopped Kalamata olives
- Salt and Black pepper to taste
- ¼ cup Olive oil
- 2 tbsps Apple cider vinegar
- 2 tbsps Lemon juice

Directions

- In a pot with salted water, place the potatoes. Bring to a boil and cook for 20 minutes. Drain and let cool.

- Mix the olive oil, vinegar, lemon juice, and dill in a bowl.

- Add in cucumber, red onion, and olives. Toss to coat.

- Stir in the potatoes.

- Season with salt and pepper. Serve.

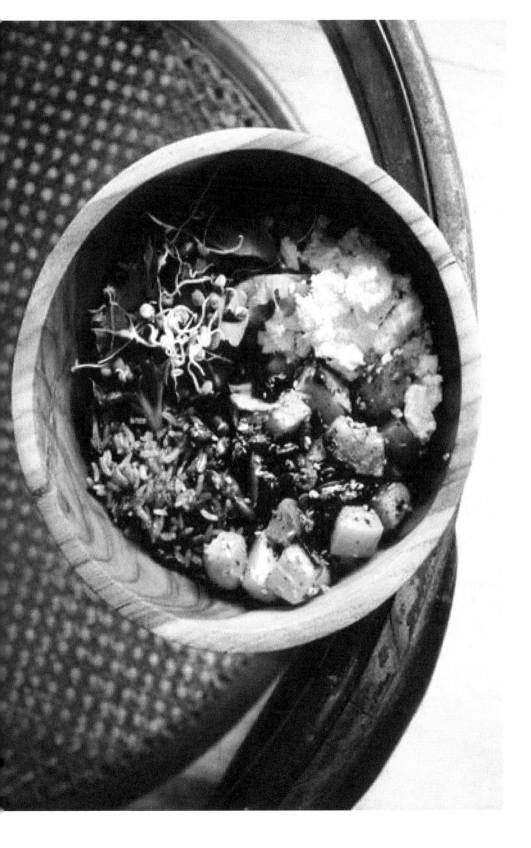

Beet & Cucumber Salad with Balsamic Dressing

4 Servings

Preparation time: 40 minutes

Ingredients

- 3 Beets, peeled and sliced
- 4 tbsps Balsamic dressing
- 2 tbsps chopped Almonds
- 2 tbsps chopped Almonds 1 tsp Olive oil
- 1 Cucumber, sliced
- 2 cups mixed greens

Directions

- Preheat oven to 390 F.

- In a bowl, stir the beets, oil, and salt.

- Toss to coat.

- Transfer to a baking dish and roast for 20 minutes, until golden brown.

- Once the beets are ready, divide between 2 plates and place a cucumber slice on each beet. Top with mixed greens.

- Pour over the dressing and garnish with almonds to serve.

DINNER

Black-Eyed Pea Oat Bake

6 Servings

Preparation Time: 25 minutes

Ingredients

- 1 Carrot, shredded
- ½ cup Breadcrumbs
- ¼ cup minced fresh Parsley
- 1 tbsp soy sauce
- ½ tsp dried sage
- Salt and Black pepper to taste
- 1 onion, chopped
- 2 Garlic cloves, minced
- 1 (15.5-oz) can black-eyed peas
- ¾ cup whole-wheat flour
- ¾ cup quick-cooking oats

Directions

- Preheat oven to 360 F.
- Combine the carrot, onion, garlic, and peas and pulse until creamy and smooth in a blender.
- Add in flour, oats, breadcrumbs, parsley, soy sauce, sage, salt, and pepper. Blend until ingredients are evenly mixed.
- Spoon the mixture into a greased loaf pan.
- Bake for 40 minutes until golden.
- Allow it to cool down for a few minutes before slicing. Serve immediately.

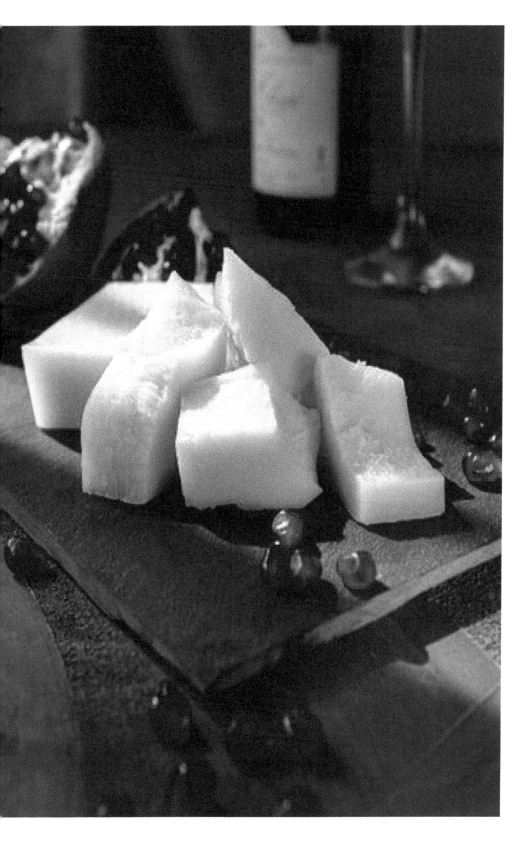

Paprika Fava Bean Patties
6 Servings

Preparation Time: 15 minutes

Ingredients
- 2 tbsps Olive oil
- 1 minced Onion
- 1 Garlic clove, minced
- 1 (15.5-oz) can fava beans
- 1 tbsp minced fresh Parsley
- ½ cup breadcrumbs
- ¼ cup almond flour
- 1 tsp smoked paprika
- ½ tsp dried thyme
- 4 burger Buns, toasted
- 4 lettuce Leaves
- 1 ripe Tomato, sliced

Directions
- In a blender, add onion, garlic, beans, parsley, breadcrumbs, flour, paprika, thyme, salt, and pepper.
- Pulse until uniform but not smooth.
- Shape 4 patties out of the mixture. Refrigerate for 15 minutes.
- Heat olive oil in a pan over medium heat.
- Fry the patties for 10 minutes on both sides until golden brown. Serve in toasted buns with lettuce and tomato slices.

Walnut Lentil Burgers

6 Servings

Preparation Time: 70 minutes

Ingredients

- 2 tbsps Olive oil
- ½ cup Walnuts
- 1 tbsp Tomato puree
- ¾ cup Almond flour
- 2 tsps curry powder
- 4 whole-grain buns
- 1 cup dry lentils, rinsed
- 2 Carrots, grated
- 1 Onion, diced

Directions

- Put lentils in a pot and cover them with water. Bring to a boil and simmer for 15-20 minutes.

- Meanwhile, combine the carrots, walnuts, onion, tomato puree, flour, curry powder, salt, and pepper in a bowl. Toss to coat.

- Once the lentils are ready, drain and transfer them into the veggie bowl.

- Mash the mixture until sticky. Shape the mixture into balls; flatten to make patties.

- Heat the oil in a skillet over medium heat. Brown the patties for 8 minutes on both sides.

- To assemble, put the cakes on the buns and top with your desired toppings.

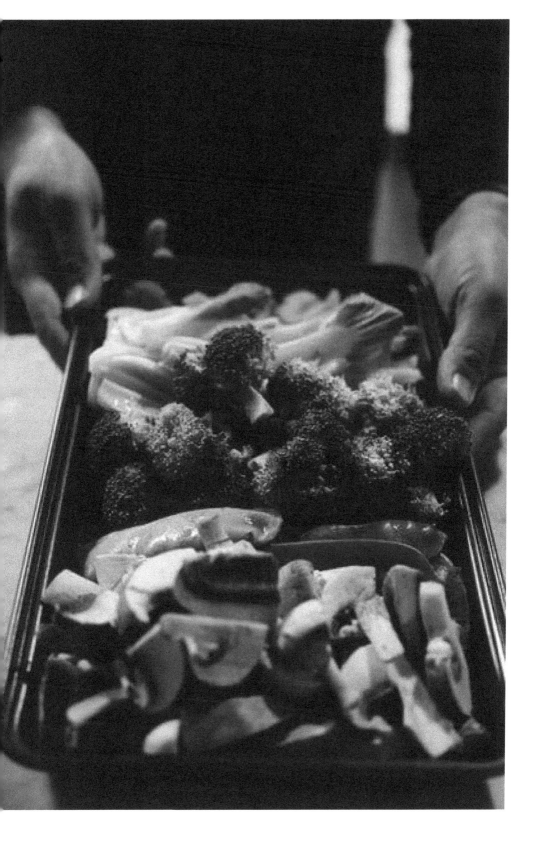

Couscous & Quinoa Burgers
6 Servings

Preparation Time: 20 minutes

Ingredients

- 2 tbsps olive oil
- ½ tsp garlic powder
- Salt to taste
- 4 burger buns
- Lettuce leaves, for serving
- Tomato slices, for serving
- ¼ cup couscous
- ¼ cup boiling water
- 2 cups cooked quinoa
- 2 tbsps balsamic vinegar
- 3 tbsps chopped olives

Directions

- Preheat oven to 350 F.

- In a bowl, place the couscous with boiling water. Let sit covered for 5 minutes.

- Once the liquid is absorbed, fluff with a fork.

- Add in quinoa and mash them to form a chunky texture. Stir in vinegar, olive oil, olives, garlic powder, and salt.

- Shape the mixture into 4 patties.

- Arrange them on a greased tray and bake for 25-30 minutes.

- To assemble, place the patties on the buns and top with lettuce and tomato slices. Serve.

Bean & Pecan Sandwiches
6 Servings

Preparation Time: 20 minutes

Ingredients

- 1 onion, chopped
- Salt and black pepper to taste
- ½ tsp ground sage
- ½ tsp sweet paprika
- 2 tbsps olive oil
- Bread slices
- Lettuce leaves and sliced tomatoes
- 1 garlic clove, crushed
- ¾ cup pecans, chopped
- ¾ cup canned black beans
- ¾ cup almond flour
- 2 tbsps minced fresh parsley
- 1 tbsp soy sauce
- 1 tsp Dijon mustard + to serve

Directions

- Add the onion, garlic, and pecans in a blender and pulse until roughly ground. Add in the beans and pulse until everything is well combined.

- Shift it to a large mixing bowl and stir in the flour, parsley, soy sauce, mustard, salt, sage, paprika, and pepper.

- Mold patties out of the mixture.

- Heat the oil in a pan over medium heat. Brown the patties for 10 minutes on both sides.

- To assemble, lay patties on the bread slices and top with mustard, lettuce, and tomato slices.

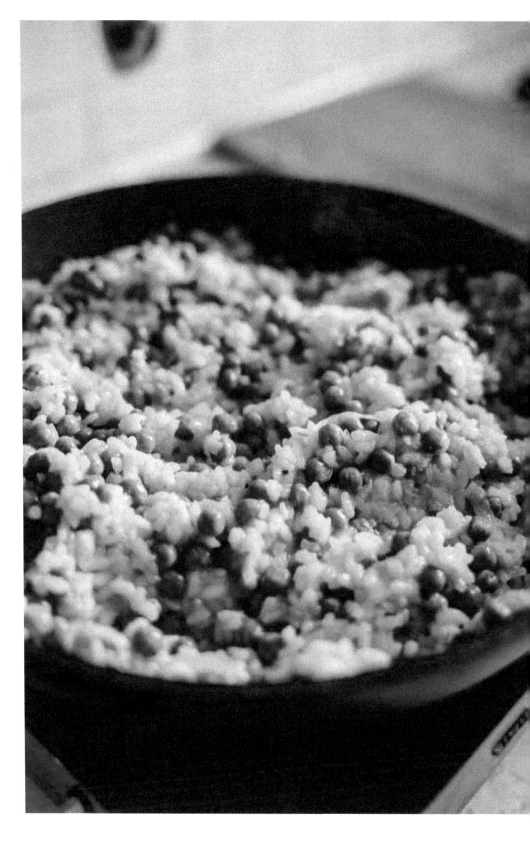

Homemade Kitchari

6 Servings

Preparation time: 40 minutes

Ingredients

- 4 cups chopped Cauliflower and broccoli florets
- ½ tsp ground Ginger
- 1 tsp ground Turmeric
- 1 tsp Olive oil
- 1 tsp fennel seeds
- Juice of 1 large Lemon
- Salt and black pepper to taste
- ½ cup split peas
- ½ cup brown rice
- 1 red onion, chopped
- 1 (14.5-oz) can diced tomatoes
- 3 garlic cloves, minced
- 1 jalapeño pepper, seeded

Directions

- In a blender, place the onion, tomatoes with juices, garlic, jalapeño pepper, ginger, turmeric, and 2 tbsps of water.

- Pulse until ingredients are evenly mixed.

- Heat the oil in a pot over medium heat.

- Cook the cumin and fennel seeds for 2-3 minutes, stirring often.

- Pour in the puréed mixture, split peas, rice, and 3 cups of water.

- Bring to a boil, then lower the heat and simmer for 10 minutes.

- Stir in cauliflower, broccoli, and cook for another 10 minutes. Mix in lemon juice and adjust seasoning.

Sauté Quinoa

6 Servings

Preparation Time: 30 minutes

Ingredients

- 1 cup Quinoa
- 2 Scallions, chopped
- 2 tbsps Water
- 1 tsp toasted Sesame oil
- 1 tbsp Soy sauce
- 2 tbsps Sesame seeds
- Salt to taste
- 1 head Cauliflower, break into florets
- 2 tsps untoasted Sesame oil
- 1 cup snow Peas, cut in half
- 1 cup frozen peas
- 2 cups chopped Swiss chard

Directions

- Put quinoa with 2 cups of water and salt in a bowl. Bring to a boil, lower the heat and simmer for 15 minutes. Do not stir.

- Heat the oil in a skillet over medium heat and sauté the cauliflower for 4-5 minutes. Add in snow peas and stir well. Stir in Swiss chard, scallions, and 2 tbsps of water; cook until wilted, about 5 minutes. Season with salt.

- Drizzle with sesame oil and soy sauce and cook for 1 minute. Divide the quinoa into bowls and top with the cauliflower mixture. Garnish with sesame seeds and soy sauce to serve.

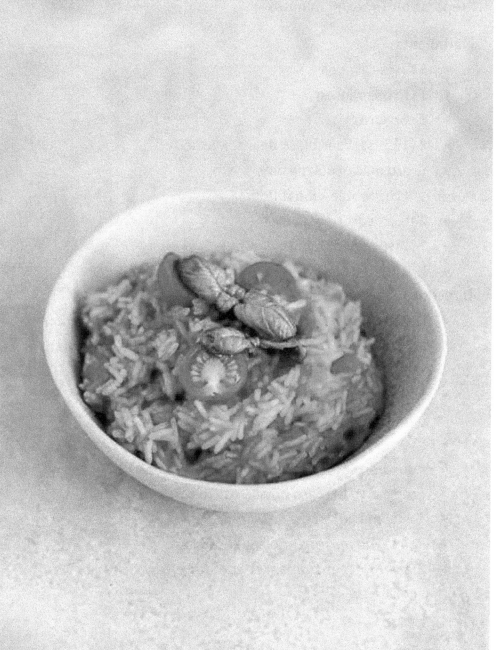

Faro & Black Bean Loaf

6 Servings

Preparation Time: 40 minutes

Ingredients

- 3 tbsps Olive oil
- 1 Onion, minced
- 1 cup faro
- 2 (15.5-oz) cans black beans, mashed
- ½ cup quick-cooking oats
- 1/3 cup whole-wheat flour
- 2 tbsps nutritional yeast
- 1 ½ tsps dried thyme
- ½ tsp dried oregano

Directions

- Heat the oil in a pot over medium heat. Place in onion and sauté for 3 minutes. Add in faro, 2 cups of water, salt, and pepper.
- Bring to a boil, lower the heat and simmer for 20 minutes. Remove to a bowl.
- Preheat oven to 350 F.
- Add the mashed beans, oats, flour, yeast, thyme, and oregano to the faro bowl. Toss to combine.
- Taste and adjust the seasoning.
- Shape the mixture into a greased loaf.
- Bake for 20 minutes. Let cool for a few minutes. Slice and serve.

DESSERT

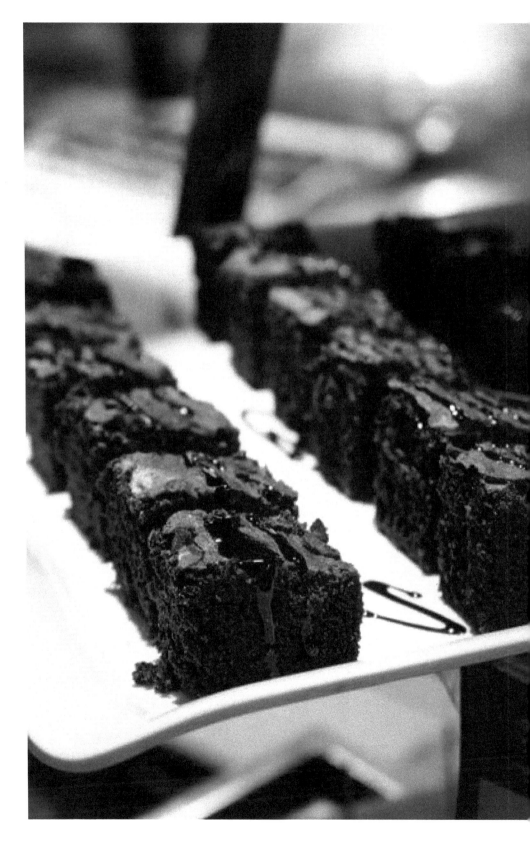

Vegan Brownies

4 Servings

Preparation Time: 30 minutes

Ingredients

- 2 tbsps flaxseed powder
- ¼ cup cocoa powder
- ½ cup almond flour
- ½ tsp baking powder
- ½ cup erythritol
- 10 tablespoons plant butter
- 2 oz dairy-free dark chocolate
- ½ teaspoon vanilla extract

Directions

- Preheat oven to 375 F and line a baking sheet with parchment paper. Mix the flaxseed powder with 6 tbsps water in a bowl and allow thickening for 5 minutes.
- In a separate bowl, mix cocoa powder, almond flour, baking powder, and erythritol until no lumps. In another bowl, add the plant butter and dark chocolate and melt both in the microwave for 30 seconds to 1 minute.
- Whisk the vegan "flax egg" and vanilla into the chocolate mixture, and then pour the mixture into the dry ingredients. Combine evenly.
- Pour the batter onto the paper-lined baking sheet and bake for 20 minutes. Cool completely and refrigerate for 2 hours. When ready, slice into squares and serve.

Vegan Cheesecake with Blueberries
6 Servings

Preparation Time: 1 Hour 30 minutes

Ingredients

- 2 oz plant butter
- 1 ¼ cups almond flour
- 3 tbsps Swerve sugar
- 1 tsp vanilla extract
- 3 tbsps flaxseed powder
- 2 cups cashew cream cheese
- ½ cup coconut cream
- 1 tsp lemon zest
- 2 oz fresh blueberries

Directions

- Preheat oven to 350 F and grease a springform pan with cooking spray. Line with parchment paper.

- To make the crust, melt the plant butter in a skillet over low heat until nutty in flavor. Turn the heat off and stir in almond flour, 2 tbsps of Swerve sugar, and half of the vanilla until a dough forms. Press the mixture into the springform pan and bake for 8 minutes.

- Mix flaxseed powder with 9 tbsps water and allow sitting for 5 minutes to thicken. In a bowl, combine cashew cream cheese, coconut cream, remaining Swerve sugar, lemon zest, remaining vanilla extract, and vegan "flax egg." Remove the crust from the oven and pour the mixture on top. Use a spatula to layer evenly. Bake the cake for 15 minutes at 400 F. Then, reduce the heat to 230 F and bake for 45-60 minutes. Remove to cool completely. Refrigerate overnight and scatter the blueberries on top. Serve.

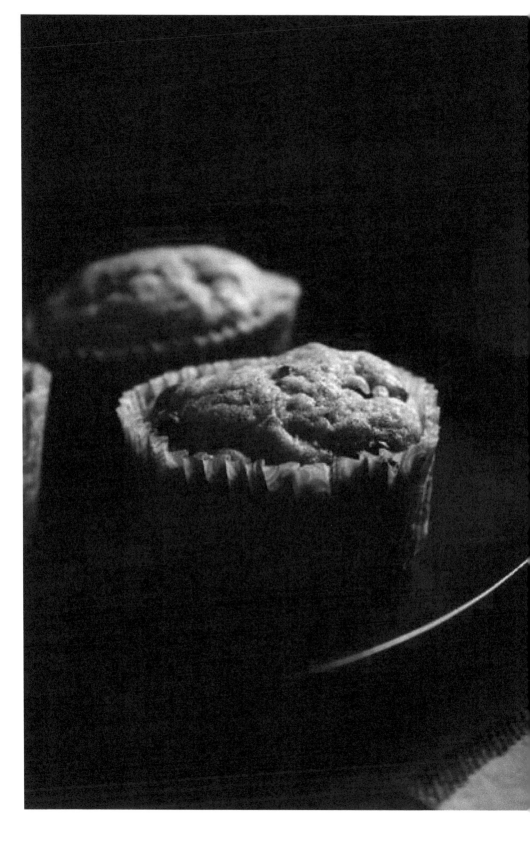

Lime Avocado Ice Cream

4 Servings

Preparation Time: 10 minutes

Ingredients

- 2 large avocados, pitted
- Juice and zest of 3 limes
- 1/3 cup erythritol
- 1 ¾ cups coconut cream
- ¼ tsp vanilla extract

Directions

- In a blender, combine the avocado pulp, lime juice and zest, erythritol, coconut cream, and vanilla extract. Process until the mixture is smooth.

- Pour the mixture into your ice cream maker and freeze based on the manufacturer's instructions. When ready, remove and scoop the ice cream into bowls.

- Serve immediately.

Vanilla White Chocolate Pudding

4 Servings

Preparation Time: 20 minutes

Ingredients

- 3 tbsps flaxseed + 9 tbsps water
- 3 tbsps cornstarch
- 1 cup cashew cream
- 2 ½ cups almond milk
- ½ pure date sugar
- 1 tbsp vanilla caviar
- 6 oz white chocolate chips
- Whipped coconut cream
- Sliced bananas and raspberries

Directions

- In a small bowl, mix the flaxseed powder with water and allow thickening for 5 minutes to make the vegan "flax egg." In a large bowl, whisk the cornstarch and cashew cream until smooth. Beat in the vegan "flax egg" until well combined.

- Pour the almond milk into a pot and whisk in the date sugar.

- Cook over medium heat while frequently stirring until the sugar dissolves. Reduce the heat to low and simmer until steamy and bubbly around the edges.

- Pour half of the almond milk mixture into the vegan "flax egg" mix, whisk well and pour this mixture into the remaining milk content in the pot.

- Whisk continuously until well combined. Bring the new mixture to a boil over medium heat while still frequently stirring and scraping all the pot's corners, 2 minutes.

- Turn the heat off, stir in the vanilla caviar, then the white chocolate chips until melted. Spoon the mixture into a bowl, allow cooling for 2 minutes, cover with plastic wraps, making sure to press the plastic onto the surface of the pudding, and refrigerate for 4 hours.

- Remove the pudding from the fridge, take off the plastic wrap, and whip for about a minute. Spoon the dessert into serving cups, swirl some coconut whipping cream on top, and top with the bananas and raspberries. Enjoy.

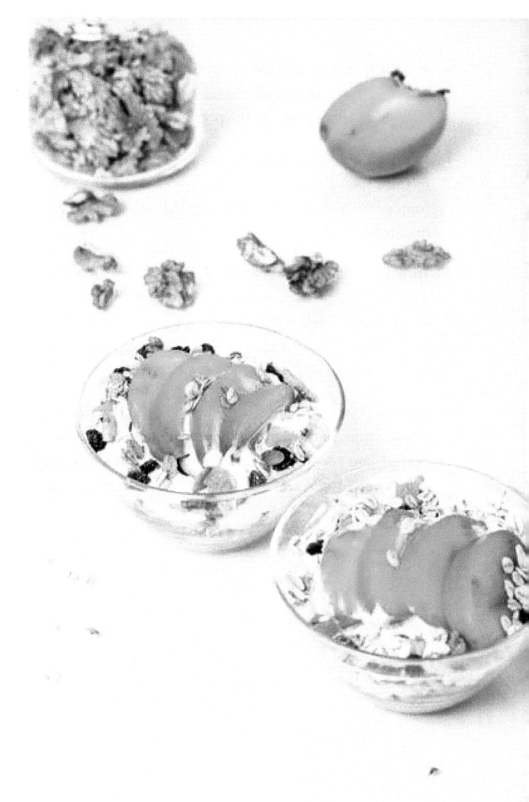

Apricot Tarte Tatin

4 Servings

Preparation Time: 30 minutes

Ingredients

- 4 tbsps flaxseed powder
- ¼ cup almond flour
- 3 tbsps whole-wheat flour
- ½ tsp salt
- ¼ cup cold plant butter, crumbled
- 3 tbsps pure maple syrup
- 4 tbsps melted plant butter
- 3 tsps pure maple syrup
- 1 tsp vanilla extract
- 1 lemon, juiced
- 12 apricots, halved and pitted
- ½ cup coconut cream
- 4 fresh basil leaves

Directions

- Preheat the oven to 350 F and grease a large pie pan with cooking spray.

- In a medium bowl, mix the flaxseed powder with 12 tbsps water and allow thickening for 5 minutes.

- In a large bowl, combine the flours and salt. Add the plant butter, and using an electric hand mixer, whisk until crumbly. Pour in the vegan "flax egg" and maple syrup and mix until smooth dough forms.

- Flatten the dough on a flat surface, cover with plastic wrap, and refrigerate for 1 hour.

- Dust a working surface with almond flour, remove the dough onto the surface, and using a rolling pin, flatten the dough into a 1-inch diameter circle. Set aside.

- In a large bowl, mix the plant butter, maple syrup, vanilla, and lemon juice. Add the apricots to the mixture and coat well.

- Arrange the apricots (open side down) in the pie pan and lay the dough on top. Press to fit and cut off the dough hanging on the edges.

- Brush the top with more plant butter and bake in the oven for 35 to 40 minutes or until golden brown and puffed up.

- Remove the pie pan from the oven, allow cooling for 5 minutes, and run a butter knife around the edges of the pastry.

- Invert the dessert onto a large plate, spread the coconut cream on top, and garnish with the basil leaves. Slice and serve.

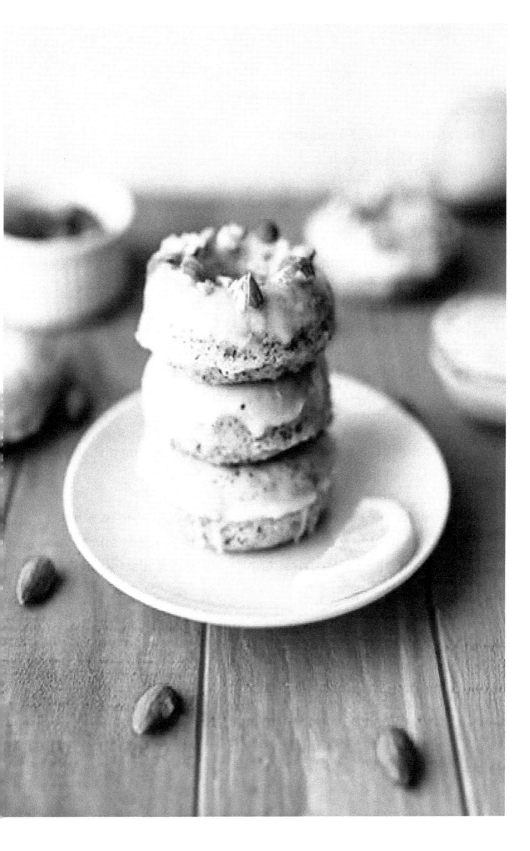

Southern Apple Cobbler with Raspberries
4 Servings

Preparation Time: 50 minutes

Ingredients

- 3 apples, chopped
- 2 tbsps pure date sugar
- 1 cup fresh raspberries
- 2 tbsps unsalted plant butter
- ½ cup whole-wheat flour
- 1 cup toasted rolled oats
- 2 tbsps pure date sugar
- 1 tsp cinnamon powder

Directions

- Preheat the oven to 350 F and grease a baking dish with some plant butter.

- Add apples, date sugar, and 3 tbsps of water to a pot. Cook over low heat until the date sugar melts and then mix in the raspberries. Cook until the fruits soften, 10 minutes.

- Pour and spread the fruit mixture into the baking dish and set aside.

- In a blender, add the plant butter, flour, oats, date sugar, and cinnamon powder. Pulse a few times until crumbly.

- Spoon and spread the mixture on the fruit mix until evenly layered. Bake in the oven for 25 to 30 minutes or until golden brown on top. Remove the dessert; allow cooling for 2 minutes, and serve.

CPSIA information can be obtained
at www.ICGtesting.com
Printed in the USA
LVHW021537110521
687091LV00003B/281